HOW TO

MEN

THE RIGHT WAY

The Only 7 Steps You Need to Master What Men Want, Attraction Techniques and How to Pick Up Today

Dean Mack

© **Copyright 2018 by Dean Mack. All rights reserved.**

This document is geared towards providing exact and reliable information in regards to the topic and issue covered. The publication is sold with the idea that the publisher is not required to render accounting, officially permitted, or otherwise, qualified services. If advice is necessary, legal or professional, a practiced individual in the profession should be ordered.

From a Declaration of Principles which was accepted and approved equally by a Committee of the American Bar Association and a Committee of Publishers and Associations.

In no way is it legal to reproduce, duplicate, or transmit any part of this document in either electronic means or in printed format. Recording of this publication is strictly prohibited and any storage of this document is not allowed unless with written permission from the publisher. All rights reserved.

The information provided herein is stated to be truthful and consistent, in that any liability, in terms of inattention or otherwise, by any usage or abuse of any policies, processes, or directions contained within is the solitary and utter responsibility of the recipient reader. Under no circumstances will any legal responsibility or blame be held against the publisher for any reparation, damages, or monetary loss due to the information herein, either directly or indirectly.

Respective authors own all copyrights not held by the publisher.

The information herein is offered for informational purposes solely, and is universal as so. The presentation of the information is without contract or any type of guarantee assurance.

The trademarks that are used are without any consent, and the publication of the trademark is without permission or backing by the trademark owner. All trademarks and brands within this book are for clarifying purposes only and are the owned by the owners themselves, not affiliated with this document.

Table of Contents

Table of Contents 4

Introduction 5

Chapter One - Step One: The Body Language of Seduction ... 9

Chapter Two - Step Two: Secrets of Dating Online 20

Chapter: Three – Step Three: Talk the Talk 30

Chapter Four – Step Four: Go Flirt Happy Girl 38

Chapter Five - Step Five: The Seduction Game 48

Chapter Six – Step Six: How to Get Him Crazy in Bed 59

Chapter Seven – Step Seven: Keep Your Man Hooked and Happy 64

Conclusion 70

Introduction

Are you having trouble attracting the man of your dreams? Do you want to be the ultimate man magnet who always gets the most attractive, intelligent, successful, and understanding men? There's a piece of good news and bad news – the bad news is that there is not shortcut to getting the best men.

The good news, however, is that it isn't an impossible task. A man's brain is wired differently from a woman's. The psyche, thoughts, and emotions are all processed differently. Their minds are mapped differently, and any success with getting the best men begins by unlocking the secret to reading/understanding their mind.

Many thoughts, feelings, and situations will be interpreted in dramatically different ways because of the differences in the way men and woman think. When you have the key to understanding what exactly a man seeks, your chances of attracting their attention and forming fulfilling relationships increases. You get a considerable edge over others who don't understand the secret to unlocking their way through a man's heart. When you know practical, workable and effective solutions to make your way into a man's heart, it doesn't stop you from getting any man you want.

There are complex dynamics involved in the evolution of the human species, which helps you put together the puzzle of what a man truly wants in a woman. There are multiple evolutionary, psychological and neurological secrets involved in attracting the right man. Use these scientific secrets to your advantage by understanding precisely what a man wants.

For example, as a lady, won't you be more attracted to a man who is positive, healthy and boasts of healthy testosterone levels? Now, throw in a pleasantly charming personality, affectionate nature, chivalry, and a dazzling sense of humor. Wouldn't you really be attracted to a man who can be your knight in shining armor to look after you? From primordial ages, men have been hunters and gatherers, who've collected food for their family and protected them from the dangers of the jungle. This explains why until today our brains are wired to be attracted to men who are good providers and protectors. Now add to this primitive behavior the fundamental contemporary dynamics, where roles are easily interchangeable. This makes the relationship between men and women even more complicated.

Seduction, flirting and picking up isn't any less than a game, and to master any game, you need to learn its rules. I'll let you in on the secret rules, strategies and cheat-sheets involved to ace this game.

Similarly, based on the way their minds are mapped, men find certain traits highly attractive in a woman.

What you believe to be plain bad luck or lack of social skills when it comes to dating may simply be sending the wrong signals or aura that sends men away. Sometimes, without even without realizing it, we transmit the wrong vibes to people, which totally ruins our chances of enjoying fulfilling relationships.

How many times have you unfortunately wondered that a man is absolutely not in your league or totally unattainable? No one is outside your league. You can get any man you want if you have the confidence, self-belief and of course, a few amazing tricks up your sleeve. You have to tap into his subconscious mind to understand him and draw him closer to you. Yes, of course, a red lipstick, a sexy tank top, stilettos and a gorgeous smile helps, but it is all a mind game at the end of the day. If you are able to sway their subconscious mind in the right direction, you'll have them eating straight out of your palms.

The secret to making your way into a man's heart is by appealing and talking to his mind. When his subconscious mind views you as desirable, seducing, flirting and picking him up becomes a cakewalk.

There's a huge difference between men checking you out and men who just cannot keep away from your spell. Yes, the sheer magnetism where a guy can resist succumbing to your charm. This is exactly why realms of paper are being dedicated to research about attracting the opposite sex. We don't simply want men gaping at us, we want men who are hooked to us.

In the next few chapters, I will offer you the ultimate secrets for attracting the man you desire using practical and actionable tips that work in the real world. These are a combination of scientific, psychological, evolutionary and perfectly common sense tips that will open up a whole new world of dating and attracting men to you.

Chapter One -Step One: The Body Language of Seduction

For starters, conversation, pickup lines and texts can wait! Body language is the unsung superstar of dating. It isn't as much about what you are actually thinking or conveying. It's about how to make it positive enough for the other person to perceive it in a manner you intend.

Imagine having a superpower or secret weapon that can help you communicate your deepest thoughts, feelings and emotions without having to use a single word. Well, body language is indeed that superpower that helps you manipulate how others perceive you.

Research has revealed that people recall only 10 percent of the information that is passed on to them verbally and about 20 percent of the information communicated visually. However, when both verbal and nonverbal communication is combined, a staggering 80 percent of the message is absorbed.

When we keep our body language in a particular manner, we not just lead others to perceive what we want them to, but also trick our subconscious mind into believing its truth. So when you stand all tall and erect, you are actually leading your subconscious mind into believing that you are actually important and confident. The subconscious mind then directs out body to behave in a matching confident and self-assured manner. Let's just call it a little mind game you're playing with your subconscious mind.

If you combine both orally and visually communicated information, 80 percent of the information is retained.

For instance, if you want to reveal yourself as a sexy, confident seductress, your body language should help the other person perceive it without any trouble. Basically, if you're giving the wrong signals, the person will just not get it. So how does one give out the right message? Here's unlocking some of the most powerful body language secrets.

1. Smile

There are some universal gestures of acceptance and interest, and smile tops that list. You meet someone nice you truly into or interested in, shake hands, get their name, use the name and greet them with their name and finally, flash your most dazzling, hypnotizing smile. There's nothing more irresistible than a woman giving a warm, affectionate and confident smile that says, "I am ready if you are".

2. The Belly Button Rule

Your belly button should ideally face the individual you're truly attracted to. Even if you are facing the person or in another direction while talking to him, change your position to keep your belly button straight in front of the man you are interested in or addressing. It sends out a sort of subconscious message that you are totally into him, and focusing all your attention (including the body) in their direction. It works at a very primordial level. Try it!

3. The Magic Touch

Touch is the cornerstone of the dating and mating game. Even a slight touch can communicate intimacy and increase one's heart rates. It may not be a good idea to grab a man by his arm the moment you are introduced to him. However, a few flirtatious or gentle touches around a man's wrist or arm can do you a whole lot of good. This is a good first or second date strategy. Keep the frequency at a minimum of five times for every 15 minutes.

4. Stand in the Center of a Group

So if you are really looking to attract a man, stand smack in the center of your pack. You are more likely to be spotted and subconsciously viewed as a leader of the pack if you are standing in the middle rather than the outskirts. Even if you are not straightaway standing in the center, make your way into the center subtly. You are literally having yourself amed or flanked by others, and making it appear like you the group's influencer. Hey, and who doesn't love leaders influencers? Also, the human eyes are naturally drawn to people who are in the center of a space as that becomes the point of focus.

5. The Posture

Don't look hunched over that phone. Put it away now. That's not the best way to attract the attention of the man you want. Did you hear about Amy Cuddy's TED Talk research where she reveals that once you're bent, the body's cortisol level rise and testosterone level lowers? Yes, that's right. The moment you hunch, the body's stress hormones increase dramatically. No, that certainly doesn't mean you walk in with an obvious power pose or worse, exaggerated swag.

Maintain a subtle power pose by standing with your arms on the hips. The feet should ideally be about six inches away. According to research conducted by Cuddy, adopting a subtle power pose can reduce your stress level and increases testosterone levels, and make you feel even more confident and positive.

Now, why not use body language and posture to display your most flattering physical attributes? Notice how some women look amazing when they pull back their neck and shoulders and stand with their breasts out? If you have long legs, stand tall and keep ramp like sideway leg posture to demonstrate a sexy pair of legs. Reveal your best and most flattering attributes.

Sit up straight or lean back to appear more confident and flaunt your most attractive physical attributes. Want to make your butt look amazing? Arch your back and throw your shoulders behind. Bonus points if you're wearing a foxy, sexy pair of stilettos.

6. Use Hands, Duh!

One of the most effective ways to attract men is to use your hand generously, and not in the way you're thinking yet! Hint romantic actions and activities through hand gestures. It could be anything from caressing yourself to gently tapping your chest to touching your face or legs. There's no harm in dropping a little hint or being suggestive/flirtatious.

It communicates two things —something you'd like to do to the man or something that you'd like the man to do to you. If you're really creative, you can also use a bunch of props or objects to communicate the same thing. Some objects you can use include drink glasses and cigarettes. Subtle fidgeting will send powerful signals to the object of your desire about what you intend to do with them or that you have your eyes firmly fixated on them.

7. Let Your Lips Do the Talking

So what should be your first move when it's time to take control of wooing the man of your dreams? Your lips are the best 'go for the kill' weapons. Start talking to the man of your dreams. Now here's the trick, and this has to be done very subtly. Gently lick, purse or bite your lips. The lip movement should be noticeable without being in your face. You may already be doing this subconsciously. However, now be more mindful of it. Start doing it frequently while talking to the man you desire.

When you're eating, ensure you are doing it gradually, mindfully and intentionally. They will just not be able to resist your lip movements and will start sending cushy, romantic signals right back. Woohoo, you've scored a point!

8. Let Your Expressions Do the Trick

A majority of the time we think our facial expressions are a result of our subconscious actions that we have little control over. That may not be very true. If you read and learn more about body language, you realize that it can be manipulated to help the other person perceive a certain feeling or thought on a subconscious level.

Keep your expressions more engaging, involved and dramatic. Ensure you nod periodically (but not frequently enough to appear too eager to please) when the man of your dream is speaking to you. Appear enthusiastic and interested in what they are speaking. Acknowledge what they are saying with matching expressions or a nod. I'll give you a few killer tips to appear excited and interested while having a conversation with that special someone. Slowly lift your eyebrows, make consistent eye contact (yes more on this later) and mirror his expressions. It will help him connect with you on a subconscious level.

9. Mirror His Actions

As discussed in the earlier point mirroring a person's expressions, gestures, posture and body language works brilliantly on a subconscious level. Going back to evolutionary science, we instantly take to people who seem to belong to our type or kind. It had existed since primitive times when humans aped each other's actions to demonstrate their loyalty or belongingness for their tribe or group. It is referred to as a sense of affiliation in psychology, which is nothing but the motivation to belong to a certain group around us.

Today, when you mirror a person's gestures, expressions, and other body language, they receive subconscious signals that you are 'one among them,' which makes them take an instant liking for you. Be careful, however, that you don't overdo it or it will appear like you are imitating the man or worse, making fun of him. That's the last thing you want.

Keep it classy and subtle. You can hold your wine glass the way he has held his. Sip on your drink right after he takes a sip of his drink. Lean a little ahead if you find him leaning ahead while talking to you. If he is leaning against a wall, follow suit and lean subtly against a wall. Try and listen to the words he uses during the conversation very intently. Use the same words in your conversation to make yourself appear more and more like him.

Again, be discreet while mirroring his actions or you'll come across as too eager to please or without a mind of your own. Mirror his actions judiciously, but also retain your individuality.

10. Throw in Eye Contact

Of course, in the business world, continuous eye contact can be intimidating and unnerving. You'll be left wondering why the hell your associate or boss is giving you such intense looks. However, in social relationships, it works slightly differently. It conveys a sense of intimacy, interest, and attraction. It shows you are truly excited about meeting him and eager to know more about him.

Want to cast an even more effective spell on the man of your dreams? Combine meaningful eye-contact with occasional touches. Also, keep darting your eyes at his lips once in a while. It works like a charm!

My favorite tip is to combine eye contact and to lean a little forward while talking to him simultaneously. Attempt to get a little closer. If you both are seated, gently brush your leg against his without making it look forced or awkward. Another thing I often suggest is throwing your arms on the table if he is seated across the table from you. Let your arms accidentally brush against his hand.

Chapter Two - Step Two: Secrets of Dating Online

If you one of those women who is very confident of approaching Mr. Perfect in person, there's hope online. Now that we book everything from airline tickets to restaurant tables on the internet, why should it stop you from finding love online? It is a wonderful way to meet new people from varied backgrounds. Also, you establish a connection with people who share similar interests, hobbies and goals. Don't even get me started with the umpteen flirting and seduction opportunities. Yes, it's a minefield of men if you just know how to snag the most desirable ones.

Though online dating has munificent advantages, it has a downside too. There are thousands of profiles out there, and you've got it to really stand out to be noticed.Plus, there are the scams and fake profiles. How then do you make your profile and virtual persona interesting from others? Fret not, I've got you covered there. There are some neat tricks up my sleeve that works like a charm on a range of dating sites.

1. Create a Wow Profile

Even if you don't want to create a detailed and elaborate profile (though creating one will increase your chances of success), you should have a minimum of one profile picture and some fundamental details. I'll show you some secret tips for creating an attractive and well-optimized dating profile that attracts a swarm of desirable men.

For starters, always use a current profile picture. Men don't want to see how you looked 10 winters ago when you were several stones lighter. They want to see your real, honest self now. Tell me, wouldn't you be big time annoyed a guy put up a profile picture when he had a massive crop of hair on his head only to find him semi-bald when you meet? That's deception, and no one appreciates it!

Avoid using heavily filtered or doctored images. They may look great on your Instagram feed but don't belong on a dating profile. Try to keep it attractive, flirty and naughty, yet real. Quick tip: research has revealed that wearing red in your display picture helps you look more desirable. Reach out for your best red outfit in the wardrobe and go click happy! Of course, you can keep it a little revealing, sexy and flirtatious. Wear a nice dress with a flattering neckline.

Your picture probably speaks more than the written introduction. There's a lot that can be read from your posture and expression. Look your flattering best minus the deception. Opt for images that highlight your best features (everything from your gorgeous mane to dimpled smile to big eyes). Again, avoid making insanely seductive or provocative expressions. It doesn't really make you come across as classy and smart. Duck faces and pouts belong to Snapchat, avoid them here like the plague.

If you have a bunch of professionally shot pictures, I would strongly recommend using them as the extra images and not your main profile picture. Use pictures that show you in a more real and natural manner as your display picture.

You'll have the option of adding several supplementary images. Use this for adding images in different settings and from varied angles. It will offer a greater range to your persona. Add pictures that reveal your interests such as camping, fishing, playing tennis. They make you come across as a multidimensional person, who has a variety of passions. Keep the count of your supplementary images limited to 10.

2. Write a Power Packed Introduction

Ensure you mention all interests clearly, and above all don't forget to be witty, creative and original. No one likes to read hackneyed introductions about how you love meeting new people or what a romantic person you are. For example, don't simply say you love going skiing. Mention your most exciting skiing experience ever. This makes you more fun and sexier.

Similarly, everyone talks about how crazy they are about food. Write about the best meal you ever had or a memorable traditional feast you enjoyed in any part of the world. Make it seductive, specific and highly descriptive by adding details. There are a million profiles that say they love listening to music. Instead, mention the kind of music you like listening to. It gives the man who approaches you more substance or ground to start the virtual conversation.

Brag a bit but don't go overboard. Don't say you are smoking hot; let your images do the talking. Similarly, don't underplay yourself. Modesty is not a trait that'll win you many virtual admirers. Be your natural, flirty and fun self. Include a few cleverly suggestive phrases in your introduction without making it tacky.

Now, your life may have been an interesting soap opera but mentioning it here doesn't fulfill any purpose. There's no need to mention past affairs or relationships gone awry. Nix the drama, and don't present yourself as a desperate attention-seeking wimp. Men don't want drama queens. They are looking for a fun, sexy and confident woman who can take care of her emotions without appearing insecure and attention-seeking. Golden rule – never ever reveal confidential or highly personal details about yourself or your past until you can trust the person.

Also, don't make your profile an elaborate grocery list. I want someone who has the perfect large, black eyes, flattering height, Harvard graduate and more. It just makes you come across as a digger who is highly demanding and controlling. Don't make it obvious that you are looking for someone like an ex-lover. While it's alright to say you want someone fun and presentable, it isn't really wise to say you only want someone who has brown eyes, brown hair and is 5'11 inches tall.

3. Go for the Kill

Don't just set up a profile, wait for men to approach you, and then go on a replying spree. Be confident and proactive when it comes to approaching men. Quick tip: Bumble.com is a dating site where only women can approach men and not vice-versa. So, the rules are changing.

Increase your chances of getting the men you fancy by approaching them confidently. A great way to begin is by asking more open-ended questions or offering constructive comments about what's written in their profile.

You really don't have to draft Shakespeare style love notes to reveal your evolved writing skills. Write a short and snappy introduction by sounding real and natural. I know a lot of dating gurus say wait for a while before replying to someone who approaches you. Nah! It doesn't work in the fast-paced virtual dating field. People don't like to wait too much.

4. Stay Safe

First things first, no one should make you do anything that you aren't happy doing. It is alright to be clear and state upfront that you are not comfortable doing certain things or have certain dating rules.

For instance, some women don't like sharing their contact number immediately, which is a good practice. They prefer communication over a series of emails before actually talking over the phone. There are several ways to keep in touch via video chats and messengers, before meeting the man. Do what makes you comfortable. There are no rules. You make your own rules to do to safeguard your privacy. Build excitement and anticipation in the run-up to your meeting. The guy should be dying to see who you are! Use light flirting to make the wait even more exciting!

Be alert, cautious and watch out for signs that don't quite feel right. It is your responsibility to look after your safety and protect your privacy.

Always insist on picking a public place that is fairly crowded for your first meeting. As far as possible, avoid meeting someone for the first time near your residence or place of work. Similarly, I always advise women to share the contact details of their date along with the venue with a trusted friend, co-worker or family member.

Carry some non-dangerous tools like a pepper spray for safety on your first date, and always remember to split the bill. Don't come across as a gold digger who is only out to have a good time at the man's expense. It isn't very attractive for most guys trust me. Women who don't accept any obligation or favors, and come across as more independent are self-respecting can be insanely sexy for a man. Hold your head high and pick up your own tab instead of expecting the man to feed you. For the first date, don't make it an expensive affair. You don't really need a Michelin restaurant. Keep it no frills, comfortable and casual, where you can actually enjoy a conversation.

Nowadays, new agers opt for plenty of fun, offbeat activities, such as mountain climbing, cycling, and museum trips. Get to know each other, while doing fun activities together seems to be the mantra.

5. The First Date

Sit in a way that makes you come across as close to him as well as approachable. Opt for a seat where he can lay his eyes on you as soon as he enters. Be playful with hair, throw a suggestive glance in his direction and talk to someone who is near him in your sexiest voice to grab his attention without directly addressing him. Ensure again that you do it subtly and don't come across as a desperate attention seeker.

This works wonders if you do it exactly as it's intended to be done. Once every few minutes, find something that keeps you looking slightly busy. It can be browsing on your phone or a leaflet/menu. Appear a little unavailable. When you look at him, he's most likely gazing in your direction. Return his gaze. Maintain eye contact for a couple of seconds, followed by soft blinking of the eyes and flashing your best smile. Then, look away. This will make him want to start a conversation right away to know more about you.

Some guys don't like breaking the ice or making the first move. Don't be shy about taking the lead here and make your first move. Simply go up to him or if he comes up to you, make eye contact and say a courteous hello. Next, ask him an open-ended question or pay him a nice compliment. Go ahead and offer a brief introduction. Keep the questions uncomplicated and interesting. What dish would you highly recommend at this eatery? Keep compliments understated, cool and casual. However, make it clear you dig him (if you really do that is).

6. Post First Date

An attractive woman is someone who doesn't forget to thank her date for the wonderful company. If you are keen on meeting him again, don't be afraid to mention it. Sometimes, he may want to see you again but a wee bit hesitant to approach you because he may not know what you are thinking. Avoid playing the guessing game, and be honest about your desire to see them again. If you don't wish to see someone again, send them a short message about how nice they are, but it didn't really click for you. End by wishing them well in their quest for finding a date. Forget the three-day cooling off period rule, and call them the next day to find out if they are truly interested in taking it further.

Chapter: Three – Step Three: Talk the Talk

Alright, so maybe by now you've managed to grab their attention or interest. Here comes the tricky part. How do you now sustain their interested and keep them hooked on your conversation skills? Just how do you seduce, attract, and pick-up a man with your words before you get to the real action? Again, you've got help! Here are some proven tips for making stellar conversation with a man to appear more fun, sexy and attractive to him.

What's Your Style?

There's no need to try hard to be something you are clearly not just to please the man. Your cover will be blown sooner or later. Each of us has our own set of strengths, which should be used smartly for keeping a man captivated. What's your style? Are you gregarious and quick-witted? Or more subtle, soft-spoken, and elegant?

Go with your inherent personality and gut feeling while striking a conversation with a man you desire. Keep in mind the setting, situation, and environment. You'll know what works and what doesn't, which will help you to keep improving upon your techniques.

Act Familiar

Even if you haven't interacted with him before, don't appear distant or like strangers. Instead be warm, comfortable and friendly around the object of your desire. Start a casual conversation as if you know each other for long. Men like women who are fun, relaxed and at ease rather than those who are innately conscious about themselves.

Stand in front of the mirror and examine how you look when you talk. Speak in a balanced, even and friendly tone with fairly spaced out speed that you use when talking to your friends. Listen mindfully to how you actually sound and the gestures you make while having a conversation. Try to talk in the same tone and speed when you are around the object of your fancy.

Don't act crazy fascinated or awe-struck by the man. There are few things that put off men as women who go out of the way to please them. They like women who keep their own personality and interests going rather than trying too hard to please. Stay engaging without appearing too eager. There's nothing more charming than a woman who knows how to be her own person. This confidence makes you terribly sexy and desirable and draws him even more to you. When you feel yourself acting like a giddy-headed, love-struck teenager, shift your gaze away from him. Avoid eye contact at such times because you reallydon't want to appear clingy.

Reveal Your Wit and Awesome Sense of Humor

Guys really dig women with a fantastic sense of humor. Find something around you to make a hilarious comment. Stick to light-hearted banter and breezy topics. Don't make a mockery of yourself by playing out the soap opera of your life, much to the amusement of your crush or date. Guys love a playful woman, and quickly bond with women who can keep it fun and humorous.

It takes a huge amount of pressure off the guy's shoulder when you take control of the conversation. He doesn't think the onus of having good time rests upon him alone. This also lightens the mood for him and makes him join in the fun. Of course, not all of us are stand-up comedians reincarnated. Practice using a few funny lines with friends (but please don't make them sound rehearsed) and check their reaction. Be funny by exaggerating things around you or happening in your life.

Appear Open and Interested

Practice active listening while conversing with the man of your dreams. Maintain eye contact, smile flirtatiously and frequently nod to show interest and enthusiasm. Ask interesting questions about what he is saying to show him that you are truly listening to him. Paraphrase the important bits or highlights of his conversation. People totally dig you when they know you care to listen to what they are saying.

Be transparent about your intentions. If you are simply looking for a casual fling or hook-up, let him know that. Similarly, if you are seeking a more long-term and fulfilling relationship, drop hints about that too. Don't appear completely absorbed and besotted by him.

Most importantly, you'll be able to pick up a lot of clues about the type of person he is through his words. It is easy to understand a person's vibe or aura simply by tuning in carefully to what they are saying. Is he the kind who will lead a conversation? Or will he simply sit back and enjoy you taking center stage? Depending on his comfort level, talk or let him do the talking.

Don't behave in an exaggerated manner and laugh at every joke he cracks or gives over the top responses to everything he says in your bid to please him. Space out or even out your reactions a bit, and make them appear more natural and not contrived or forced.

The Ice Breaker

So you see this absolutely drop dead gorgeous guy at the bar, and don't want to wait for him to come and make a conversation. How do you approach the dude? Yes, there are many fabulous pick-up lines that wonder well, but this one seldom fails. Just go near him and tell you, you smell incredibly good. What fragrance are you wearing?

Most men will be glad that you noticed them. Further, complimenting them is like the icing on the cake, they'll be truly flattered. Bonus points, if you can follow it up with something really funny, such as "I went sniffing around here a couple of times because you smelled so good." He'll most likely laugh, and that'll break the ice for further conversation. Who doesn't love a little bit of ego pampering that sounds genuine?

Similarly, if you are both at a party, you can approach him and ask him how he knows the host. You are basically creating a subconscious feeling that there is something in common between the two of you. He'll also know you must be amazing or the common friend wouldn't really be friends with you in the first place. It's like a mutual friends' test. When you see a mutual friend on Facebook, you are likelier to add that person to your friend because in your mind they've already sort of cleared the test by being your friend's friend. It works the same way.

If you are at a restaurant or coffee shop, you may want to compliment him on an accessory (watch never goes wrong, I tell ya) and ask him about it pretending that you've been picked by your office team to buy one as a gift for a co-worker. Watches are to men, what bags and probably stilettos are for a woman. They can never have enough compliments on their watch. You're calling out to their amazing taste in watches, and seeking advice on what you should buy for a co-worker. Bingo! You've hit the jackpot with a bonus of exchanging contact information to get more guidance about purchasing watches. Tralalala!

Trust me when I say this, men are really flattered when you seek their expertise or onion about something. They love to flaunt their knowledge. Even when it comes to something as recommendations from the menu or the type of coffee you should be guzzling, this is one thing that can get them started and going on a positive note. You'll win plenty of brownie points.

At the gym, you may want to ask your potential knight in shining how to use a particular machine or equipment. Men love to show off their expertise and help out whenever needed. This is also the perfect excuse for buying a coffee or protein shake for him to thank him for his training. Take it up from there. Don't forget to make your moves foxier and sexier when he's around, while still focusing on your workout.

If you spot a hottie at a concert, break the ice by asking him how many times he's seen these awesomely talented people performing. If he's totally into them, you'll have a lot in common to talk about. However, even if he hates them and has been dragged to the show, he'll have an interesting backstory to it, which can be a great conversation starter or icebreaker.

Chapter Four – Step Four: Go Flirt Happy Girl

If you're the coy, shy girl type, it may seem like a virtually impossible task to flirt with a man. However, it's much simpler than you actually imagine it to be if you make the right moves. Flirting without actually looking like you're flirting is an art to be mastered. You can rely on an approachable body language, coy gestures, a dazzling smile, light touching, suggestive touching and much more to go flirthappily with the guy of your dreams. There's a lot of flirting you can do via text messages too. Here are some smooth tricks to help you become the ultimate flirt magnet.

Setting the Stage

Girls bear in mind that a guy adores being flirtedwith. Yes, they may not make it obvious or flirt outrageously. But they dig the idea of flirting. It depends on the subtle verbal and non-verbal signals you give them. If your body language is suggestive and seductive, it indicates to them at a subconscious level that you're ready for the flirting game

Let a man know you are warm, friendly and approachable if you want to flirt with him. You are the girl who doesn't really indulging in some well-meaning, flirtatious actions. Men will think a million times before trying to flirt with a woman who appears all prudish and off the limits.

Blush and Be All Coy

Guys love women who are positive, bright and happy. I'll let you in on a secret between you and me – men dig women who smile and laugh a lot while talking to them. Don't appear rude or arrogant when you're with someone you intend to flirt with. Guys run miles away from women who try to be cocky even if they are desirable looking.

Be inviting and warm when talking to your crush. Smile, blush and act coy when he compliments you or says something nice about you. He will do a mini mental dance that his compliment has had the desired effect on you.

Compliment Him Duh

Like I said earlier, guys love to be complimented. It is setting the stage for a flirt happy talk. When you like something about a person, compliment them generously about it. He will adore the fact that you actually noticed a nice thing, and more often than not he'll return the compliment and start having a flirty conversation. When he is being courteous, respectful and chivalrous, thank him for it with an affectionate smile.

When a man's chivalry is appreciated or given a more positive response, he will be even more driven to extend his courtesy and chivalry in your direction. He'll likely be even more warm, open and affectionate.

Drown In His Eyes

One of the biggest secrets of flirting is to do what people generally do when they are head over heels in love with each other. Even though you aren't there already, you don't really have to wait until you get there. Just look excited and happy in his company, and he'll be more than floored.

Next time you talk to a guy you really dig, look straight into his eyes (deeply and intensely) and offer your best smile when he's speaking. It may just end up perplexing him slightly the sight of you staring at him and smiling. However, that'll make him weak in the knees nevertheless. You're connecting at a very sensual level, where you're building a fantastic chemistry.

Tease Your Man

Learn to make fun of the man you fancy in pure jest. Say something like, your joke is lame or try harder Jack. Pulling him down slightly by teasing him in a non-offensive way is a great way to establish friendliness and familiarity. This is something you would do only with close friends or people you are really comfortable with.

By pulling his leg, you are conveying a sense of familiarity. Stay in control of the flirting game by making fun of him and then placing him on a pedestal. I'll let you in on another secret. Men are insanely competitive in nature. When you tease him even playfully, he'll try harder to do something you say he cannot.

Avoid Being Brash, Arrogant and Loud

Every manly guy with a testosterone overdrive loves a feminine or womanly woman or girly girl. Of course, you don't have to be a princess walking in glass slippers. However, do your best to be feminine, soft and subtle in everything from the way you talk to the way you dress. Don't be too brash and loud in a bid to control the conversation. You may not be too happy to read this, but few things piss a guy off as much as rude, arrogant, and loud girls who go around throwing their weight.

Again, you don't have to act all school girl-ish to win the guy's heart. However, you need to (and make that need in caps if you like) make him feel that he can protect you. Through the process of evolution, men have always been hunters, gatherers, and protectors. If you really want to attract a man, you need to give him that feeling every once in a while that he is in control. Let him take the lead sometimes. Play it simple sometimes, hold on and wait for him to take the lead in flirting.

Be Crazy Expressive

I am hoping you've seen at least one episode of Nigella Lawson's show. The gal is well in her middle ages but can give any giddy-headed teenager a run for her money when it comes to making guys go weak in their knees with her flirtatious, expressive and feminine gestures. Be expressive and feminine when you're with the guy you desire.

Spend time in the mirror and work hard on your gestures and expressions. Use your feminine charm to your benefit. I'll bet you when you master this, you'll need no words to have the man on his knees. Practice fluttering your mascara laden eyelids, work hard on getting your smile right and give out tiny little bright expressions. Do this, and you'll be the goddess of all things flirty no man can ever ignore or resist.

Do you think Hollywood actresses and other celebs are born with those insanely killer expressions? It's taken lots of practice to practice those flirtatious moves. Use your feminine expressions to the hilt for completely changing the game when it comes to attracting men like a magnet. Play it up, spice your expressions and just go for the kill lady!

Look Your Best

Flirting with men becomes much easier and way more successful when you look attractive.

Give your persona an added dose of confidence by looking your flattering best. Wear flirty, feminine clothes that highlight your best physical attributes. Opt for shapes and colors that underplay the not so flattering aspects and accentuate your best physical attributes. It's not just about donning micro miniskirts, stilettos and a heavy dose of mascara. The idea is to be well groomed, practice good hygiene and give it your best shot. People are naturally drawn to attractive, confident and presentable women who know how to carry themselves.

Set your hair nicely, keep it clean and fresh smelling. Use a good mouthwash to keep your mouth smelling great. Do your nails. Wear clean, washed and ironed clothes. A nice, well-fitting dress or skirt in red or other bright colors adds to the dazzle and makes you instantly noticeable. Don't be afraid to wear that red lipstick. Sometimes a little make-up can go a long way in playing up your best facial features.

Don't keep the same hairstyle. Try different hairdos such as straight, curly, perm, braid and bun. Experiment with make-up to know what works best for you. Find a look that you truly enjoy putting together and one that gives you confidence. Check out different stores and online catalogs for the season's latest fashion.

Flirt With Touch

Find small excuses to gently touch your crush if you want to flirt with him. It sort of creates a sexual tension and drops a hint about your desire to take it a step ahead.

Gently touch his forearm when you both are talking. When he says something funny, react by reaching your hand out and touching his arm. Put your hand on his shoulder when he is saying something serious just to communicate your support. This is great for creating a mutual camaraderie and reveals that you are completely comfortable around him.

Accidently lean in his direction when you both are walking together. If you are prepared to move to the next level with him, simply brush your hand against his to analyze his reaction.

One sneaky trick that I highly recommend is straightening his collar. Tell him subtly that his collar is slightly crooked and then lean ahead warmly to straighten it for him. Maintain eye contact with him while straightening his collar, and say something like, now that's much better and gently move back. Observe his reaction. I am saying this several times because a man's reaction to your subtle touches will offer you plenty of insights about where you both are headed.

Other signs that you're interested in flirting with him

- Unclenched hands and uncrossed arms and legs.

- Running your fingers subtly through your hair

- Pretend to pick something gently from his jacket

- Face the object of your desire directly while talking

- Wet your lips frequently. Hey and extra points if you bite them discreetly too.

Men are of course able to identify these signs, at least on the subconscious level.

Chapter Five - Step Five: The Seduction Game

It's a well-established fact that men are intensely visual creatures. They are majorly controlled by testosterone, which gives you a brilliant opportunity to spice things up. Be the ultimate seduction ninja and temptation goddess by playing out your charm in a way that is impossible for any man to resist. Here are some quick tips that will create a run up to take you both into pleasure zone.

Feel Sexy

How do you plan to seduce the man you desire if you don't feel sexy lady? Want to look and feel sexy without trying? Here's the inside dope on the business of looking good without trying. Join the much sought after sexy club.

Have you ever taken a glance of some random stranger walking on the street and be totally blown away by the sexiness that oozes through them? We all have seen that someone and wondered why the hell hasn't they be signed for any Hollywood flick yet.

Sometimes, you'll notice that they aren't even great looking. So what makes them attractive then? Some of the sexiest folks you'll bump into aren't the prettiest. However, they are still crazy sexy.

What Makes You Sexy

-A fit, healthy and well-built shape/physique

-Good grooming

- Attractive attire

- Sexy inner garments

- Pampering yourself periodically

- Respect yourself and your body

- Enjoy life

- Feel like a sexy goddess

If you fancy being a wild seductress, feel like one. Men are innately visual beings who love boobs and butts, so play it up for them. Perfect moves that accentuate your boobs and butts, and get it right each time. Let him fall for your body. Maintain a posture where your shoulders are pushed back, and your boobs are slightly out. Similarly, walk with your butt slightly out to flaunt it in all its glory. Spice it up by wearing heels, so you get this position naturally, without trying too hard. If you have a pair of toned legs, don't forget to flaunt it.

When you feel like a sexy seductress, it reflects in the way you speak and carry yourself, which in turn attracts a man. Feed into your subconscious mind that you are indeed a sexy siren, who deserves the sexiest men around. This will influence your actions to be more seductive and appealing.

Peek a Boo Baby

Yes, tease him woman! Get his testosterones raging by playing a little peek a boo game. Wear short skirts that reveal a nice pair of thighs or opt for plunging necklines. The sexy outfits will be your highway into a man's heart or ahem anywhere else you want. Of course, you'll need to find a way to ward off all the perverts you'll end up attracting.

If you really want to seduce a man, ensure you don't bear it all and wear tastelessly skimpy clothes. If you show him everything, you aren't leaving anything to his imagination. You aren't effectually challenging his testosterone. It will end up seducing the wrong kind of men or attention. Wear something that offers a teeny-weeny bit of peek a boo without giving it all away.

It is similar to whetting someone's appetite and tempting them for going after the big meal. Offer him a generous peak of what's within too. If he is standing near you, bend down slightly to pick something from the floor or your handbag. A man's eyes dart really fast in the direction of a boob graze. Giving him an exciting preview will make him want to see the entire film.

Don't Throw Yourself at Him

Women, the golden rule for classy seduction is: *Don't ever appear desperate or throw yourself on a man.* Never ever! Again, don't be too obvious in your admiration for him. Play a little hard to get. Appear a little distracted. Find other things to capture your interest. Challenge the man to try harder by appearing distracted. He'll work doubly hard to grab your attention.

If a man gets to know you think he's really hot and into you, he'll not be driven to try hard. For a man, it's all about accomplishments, whether it's a new car, woman or fragrance. It is about acquiring things that aren't easily available or attainable. He's not likely to be enticed or seduced if you make it obvious that you are already into him. That's no fun. He doesn't have to really try hard.

There's no challenge or real achievement is getting something that is easily attainable. That's their logic. He won't be impressed when he realizes you are trying hard to grab his attention. He'll most likely play hard to get (you aren't the only one playing games here lady). For heaven's sake, don't appear trashy, classless and clingy. That's a huge red flag for any man. Turn the table cleverly. Make him chase you by laying an irresistible seduction trail.

Once every while, give him the royal ignore. Stop giving him attention and move to something else when things are going a little too smoothly between you two. Let him not get the feeling that's he's already made a wonderful impression on you. Ruffle up his insecurities by playing slightly hard to get.

Hit the Dance Floor

There's nothing more seductive than showing your crush all the right moves on a dance floor. You can move your body in a certain way to floor him right out there on the dance floor. If you can pick one place to go with a man you intend to seduce, opt to go clubbing.

Move your way around his body seductively while dancing together. Lean against him, show off your foxy moves and build sexual chemistry that's just waiting to explode later. Leave him something to think about with touches that linger.

Purposefully Stage Awkward Situations

Yes, you want the guy's heart and trousers to be full, don't you? Wink wink! The smart girl's guide to seducing a man comprises purposely creating awkward situations where you both are left in close physical proximity to each other.

Squeeze into a packed elevator with him, of course 'unknowingly.' Allow your butt to slightlybrush against his leg. If he's seated, just turn up from behind him and reach out for something that he placed on his table. Do this when he isn't looking. When the guy turns slightly to look at you, he will brush against your breasts. Tada! The trick is to rub your feminine parts against him. Don't make the moves obvious or if he gets everything on a platter, he won't really appreciate it much.

Even when you hug him to greet him, ensure your girly parts rub against him.If you don't make it obvious, he'll realize he is lucky to be able to touch you in seemingly off the limit places. Create situations where he gets an opportunity to touch you. The idea is to get his pants a wee bit tighter, so he fantasizes all the more about you.

Don't Underestimate the Power of Good Fragrance

One of the most overpowering subconscious influences that trigger a man's judgment is scent. A survey revealed that a staggering 89 percent men believe that a powerful scent boosts the attractiveness of a lady. And, hold it. About 55 percent of those men went ahead and stated they would get amorous only because they find a woman's perfume appealing.

Scent is often the most potent subconscious influencers when it comes to affecting our decision or feelings about the opposite sex. This is actually comparable at a very primordial level to the pheromones used by animals during the mating game.

Pro tip- As a woman, you can multiply your pheromone levels by using natural oils such as rose, jasmine, and ylang-ylang, which are famous for their aphrodisiac features. The guy will go into a tizzy simply by your presence.

Remember how Cleopatra welcomed Marc Anthony on a ship with scented sails? The exotic fragrance drove him to fall head over heels in love with her, so much so, he died for her. Moral of the story, use a sexy, subtle and feminine scent to seduce your man. However, ensure you don't go overboard because you don't really want to send the man on an allergic coughing fit, do you? Opt for floral, citrusy and light blends.

Apply it on the body's pulse points, on your wrists, behind the ears, on the elbow bend, right behind your knees and on the ankle's insides. Again, a little tip to make your aura even more fragrant and mysterious. Release a little perfume right in the air, while walking into it.

Make the smell synonymous with you, so the guy finds it really difficult to forget you. Our olfactory glands are closely connected with neurons associated with memory and retention, which is why certain smells instantly trigger specific memories for us. When a man can clearly associate a smell with you, he will find it virtually impossible to forget you. Let your fragrance be deeply embedded in the man's mind.

Use Messaging and Snapchat Ladies

There's no reason why you cannot seduce a man who isn't around. Plus, you'll be less intimated and bolder when you aren't doing it face to face. Send the guy sexy or proactive messages, pictures, or snapchats. Don't send overtly revealing pictures or again, you aren't leaving much for his imagination.

Let the dude know you dig him by transferring a picture of something subtle, classy and fun that doesn't border on obscene. How about you frolicking in a pool to spark his raging imagination? Get him thinking in the right direction.

Send him dirty messages that leave things to his imagination and compel him to think. For example, "I had this mad dream about you last time" or "I just saw something that reminded me of you." Always works!

How about something seemingly innocuous that's loaded with innuendos such as "I intend to blow your mind completely" Now it can imply a lot of things including a blowjob or that you are going to show him something really amazing. It creates an irresistible anticipation that is hard to match.

You'll notice that these messages aren't really sexual in nature. The objective is to get him wondering and pumping up the excitement. You are basically telling him exactly what may be music to his ears. Pro tip – send him a message that is short and snappy, and doesn't demand a reply.

Try to test his reaction by sending a few messages. If things don't go as expected, you can always cover it up "Oh! My apologies that message was meant for someone else." He'll be all the more subconsciously enraged as to why you meant it to someone else. Remember, stimulating a man's competitive streak always works wonders?

You'll wriggle your way out of an awkward situation, while stilling awakening his competitive spirit. Don't freak him out be sending really obvious and in your face messages that border more on sleaziness. Men abhor an overt display of crassness and sleaziness by a woman. They like it when you keep it fun, flirty, naughty and suggestive, but definitely not tasteless. You'll end up attracting the wrong kind of men if they are impressed with your sleaziness.

Chapter Six – Step Six: How to Get Him Crazy in Bed

Congratulations, you've finally gotten the object of your desire into bed with owing to your hard to resist charm. You diva you! Now it's time to steam things up in the bed in such a way that he just cannot resist your charms and get enough of you. There's a lot you can do by using some imagination and inspired moves.

It is time to replace ho-hum vanilla sex with steamier, spicier and more incredible acts. How about toys, flavored lubricants, and playful lingerie? Think an array of costumes and role play. Here are some ways to make the action under the sheets even more exciting.

1. Get giddier and frisker by popping a bottle of champagne in bed. You'll go back to being tipsy, don't care a damn about the world teens.

2. Light up a few fragrant candles in the background, and play soft music. The ambiance should reflect your soft and seductive mood.

3. Slow things down rather than rushing into rabid, zealous sex as soon as you hit the bed. Do things that prolong your time in the bedroom. Build tension in a manner that it leads to exploding pleasure.

4. Leaving love notes like a little bedroom treasure hunt game, where you send him chasing different clues until he discovers something that you are going to do with him that will completely blow his mind away.

5. Massages are a great run up to the actual sexual activity. Offer him gentle messages near his erogenous zones to get him wet and hard. It builds anticipation for the slowly commencing sexual activity. Ask the man to on his stomach. Apply gentle thumb pressure on his lower back. Move upwards gradually and sensually. You'll barely be able to reach his shoulders before he gets all fired up for action.

6. Set a few rules to build a high sense of anticipation. For example, you may want to spend some days necking and making out with your clothes still on. The next few days can be spent touching each other everywhere except genitals. Then, use your mouth instead of hands for giving pleasure. By the end of these few days, he'll be left with a huge arousal overflow that will be waiting to explore. It will lead to heavy-duty craving in his erogenous and pleasure zones.

7. Ditch predictability and savor an amazing sex life. Go down the unpredictable route by changing the location a bit. You don't need to be in the bedroom to make humdrum love. Get steaming on a pool table in the house or even a garage. When there are people around the two of you, lock your eyes to make love. Cast a few suggestive glances in your man's direction. Enjoy a round of foreplay and sex in the open. Making love under the open sky and reaching orgasm heaven gives him an altogether different high.

8. Keep all gadgets away from the bedroom. When you're enjoying the action in the bed, it's just the two of you. There should be nothing in between, including smartphones, blaring television sets and electronic gadgets. Focus on building the atmosphere of pleasure, excitement, and intimacy.

9. Play fantasy bowl for a nice lead-up to frenzied action later. Write your three most intense and deepest sexual fantasies that no one knows about. Get your man to follow suit by mentioning three of his most intense sexual fantasies. Collect the chits and throw it in a bowl. Shuffle the chits and pick up chits by turn. Talk explicitly about the fantasy that comes up. Both swap notes about how they want the act fulfilled. There's no sexual activity yet. You are simply talking about the fantasy. Now turn off the lights and get under the

sheets. Allow him to describe his fantasy while you throw your hands below the sheet. You both will be monstrously aroused before your guy finishes talking.

10. Play sex dice the next time you want to steam it up in the bedroom. All that is needed is a pair of fun adult dice that can be sourced from an adult store. Make two categories of love notes. On one set, mention sensual body parts and on another, various actions that you'd like on those body parts. It can create an amazing array of exciting combinations when you pick one of each category. Keep it fresh, try totally different positions, and work on your intimacy.

Men adore women who take the lead, are unafraid to try new things and open to a variety of experiences. They love an adventurous, exciting and proactive gal. So, don't hesitate to climb over him and get going! That's a huge-huge turn on for your man.

11. How about giving him some much needed wet pleasures? Men love action under the shower. Start by kissing each other passionately under the shower. Work up a rich lather to wash each other sensuously. It will not just leave you both smelling fresh, but also build plenty of sexual tension for the actual act to follow. How about some passionate necking and

kissing on the couch or in the dark, last row of a less crowded cinema?

12. A dirty dancing or stripping session can be the perfect prelude to several passionate, raunchy and foxy moves to follow.

13. Tie him up to the best with a pair of your sexiest stockings or leggings. Move your mouth/tongue over his erogenous zones. Place a high pillow under his head so he can clearly see all your moves and get sufficiently wet or aroused. Tease by going down on him and moving back until he cannot take it anymore.

14. Whisper sweet nothings in his ear. Few things stimulate a man's sexual drive as much as cooing softly his ears. Tell him everything you intend to do to him during your time in bed. Follow this up by kissing him lightly on the lower neck.

15. Walk around the house wearing racy underwear and a sexy pair of stilettos. This is another little gem that works like magic. The man will not want anything else but to see you strut around making sexy moves that are bound to send his testosterones gushing.

Chapter Seven – Step Seven: Keep Your Man Hooked and Happy

Now that you've got him, how do you keep him happily hooked and addicted to you? It takes more than just romantic and gestures to have him eating out of your hands and obeying everything you say. Here are some of the most powerful tips to have a man completely wrapped around your little finger.

1. Praise him publically. Few things are more effective when it comes to boosting your guy's ego than appreciating him openly in front of people. He'll feel a huge surge of gratitude and affection for you. Men love women who stand by then, believe in their abilities and support them. Do this, and he'll melt faster than wax.

2. Keep him feeling secure. Men have oversized egos, there's no denying this. The flipside, their egos are also extremely fragile. They are territorial by nature and feel easily threatened. Keep them secure in the right manner, and they'll adore you for it. Let him know that you are his if you are truly a committed and mutually exclusive couple.

3. Surprise him once in a while. Really now, it isn't solely a man's domain to buy you expensive gifts, chocolates, and flowers. Of course, you love to be pampered but so does he. Buy him something that he has been eyeing for long but hasn't got around to buy. These little surprise gifts will speak volumes about your thoughtfulness and affection for him. It'll also convey to him that you aren't simply a gold digging receiver by also someone who cares to give. Make him feel like he is indeed the luckiest man on earth to have someone like you in his life.

4. Don't let go of your inner child. Seriously, as much as men prefer a matured and in control woman, they always love someone who is a free spirit and hasn't lost touch with her inner child. A woman who is spontaneous, fun and radiates a childlike enthusiasm is fun and easy to be. She takes the stress and burdens off a man's shoulder. This is exactly why a wise person once said, "be a girl at heart and a woman in spirit." Most women mother their men and get annoyed the man behaves childishly.

Instead of behaving like a nag, simply join in the fun once in a while and act like crazy kids. He'll love that you are not playing his mother or class monitor all the time. Let him be comfortable revealing his child side in front of you. He'll love you for it.

5. Food is the fastest route to man's heart, yes! On the face of it, they'll say your cooking skills don't really matter to them. Give him a gastronomy orgasm every once in a while by whipping up his favorite meal. He'll be hopelessly hooked. Make a reservation at his favorite restaurant when you know he's busy with work and hasn't had the opportunity to dine there for long. Invest time and effort on special occasions to come up with a delicious, home-made meal. He'll appreciate the thoughtfulness and effort behind the act.

6. Seek his expert counsel, emotional support or help. A man loves to be your knight in shining armor. He wants to know that he is useful and valuable in your life. When you seek his help and counsel every now and then, his position as a problem solves is reinforced. He feels a sense of delight in making life easy for you. When you are feeling low, drained and helpless, simply walk into his arms for him to comfort you. He will be overwhelmed by the fact that he is making you feel slightly better in the middle of all that stress.

7. Avoid emasculating him. Don't belittle him or make him feel less of a man when he's made a mistake, especially in public. It doesn't help to show him down. Men don't like to be told they are wrong straight off. If he feels less of a man with your constant putting down, he will most likely seek that validation and feeling of manliness from elsewhere.

8. Don't stop dating him or flirting with him. Just because you are a couple now doesn't mean you stop doing all the fun things. Keep the passion in your relationship alive by trying fun, new things together. Plan creative dates, don't hesitate to try novel adventures/activities together and go discover different places. Pinch his butt for naughty fun or brush your hand against his thigh playfully. Don't forget to indulge in a wee bit of sexting throughout the day.

9. Be open. Thisapplies to plenty of things that you would together, including trying a new eatery in town or a new move in the bedroom. Each person has varied tastes, and to keep it interesting and exciting, you've got to keep a flexible and non-judgmental mind. As long as something doesn't hurt or is against your morals/ethics, give it a go if he likes it. Even if you want to refuse something, do it politely and diplomatically without offending him.

10. Avoid using sex as an exchange chip. Don't withhold sex because he didn't do the dishes or refused to go out with your friends. Making it a bartering chip takes its toll on the act, and ultimately your relationship. He will most likely believe that sex is just another chore or weapon rather than a pleasurable activity for you. Eventually, constant bartering will take a toll on your man, and he'll be looking for pleasure elsewhere.

11. Avoid saying unflattering things behind his back. All couples have their share of conflicts and challenges. Unless he is doing something that is unlawful or being physically/mentally abusive (in these cases you should surely seek counseling and legal help), spare your relationship the drama by involving other people in it. Don't go on a ranting spree with your family and friends. Discussing your couple problems with others can often make it worse.

12. Make your man a priority. Take the time and effort to let him know he's craved for and special even after you get him. Don't just snag him as just another acquisition and take him for granted once he is yours. Despite a busy schedule and other commitments, ensure you make time for him. It can be anything from booking tickets to watch his favorite game to sending him an affectionate text message during the day to picking up a snack he loves on the way from work. Its small gestures like these that reveal you really care. He'll know he's always on the top of your mind with these thoughtful acts.

13. Don't be an attention seeking diva. Men don't fancy drama queens and attention seeking divas. Sooner or later, they'll get tired of your shenanigans and dump you for someone who is calm, comfortable and in control. Yes, wanting his attention is alright but going to the extreme end of the spectrum regularly to be a whine queen is a different

game altogether. Attention-grabbing tactics are not seductive; they are annoying, stressful and desperate. Don't seek constant validation and attention from others. Forcing attention to yourself is a huge off, and make you unattractive to him.

14. Avoid being a nag. Don't create catastrophic metaphors out of unwashed dishes and wet towels on the bed. Women unknowingly annoy their partners by making a huge deal of trivial daily habits. Tone down the nag factor and overlook these things sometimes. Women often blow things up and start equating a man's habits as a measure of their love. For instance, He didn't pick up the crumbs from the table after I told him, which means he really doesn't love me. Remind him in a more gentle, affectionate, and humorous way when approaching your man for doing something or changing a habit.

Conclusion

Thank you for purchasing the book, *"How to Attract Men: The Right Way"*.

I sincerely hope you enjoyed reading it. I also hope the book was able to offer you a ton of actionable, practical, and easily applicable techniques to not just attract men but also keep them completely addicted to you.

The next step is to take action. Apply all these little-known secret strategies and wisdom nuggets to become the ultimate diva or man-guy magnet. Use all these killer secrets and psychological tricks to unlock the male mind to literally have him wrapped around your little finger.

Irrespective of where you are in the dating game currently, start applying these methods to experience a complete transformation from a socially awkward gal to one who gets the male species weak in their knees. It takes some practice and consistent efforts of course, but it's worth it to be a diva.

Here's to being a confident, desirable, interesting and fun guy magnet!

CPSIA information can be obtained
at www.ICGtesting.com
Printed in the USA
LVHW080528190922
728702LV00012B/539